CU00833449

1

Table of Contents

Introduction

The Metabolic Blowtorch Diet is a type of strategy that involves a fasting protocol meant to help with fat loss and muscle preservation. Intermittent fasting isn't anything new, but this diet takes its own direction with that concept.

What's Involved in The Metabolic Blowtorch Diet

The Metabolic Blowtorch Diet is a strategy that shifts and adapts depending on what you happen to be doing in a day. For example, the way you eat will change depending on whether it is a training day or a non-training day. There are also some differences to be observed by men and women, to be discussed later in this review.

On non-training days, intermittent fasting is a central component of the Metabolic Blowtorch Diet design. On training days, there is a focus on adjusting carbohydrate intake. This is particularly true on days when weight training is involved.

The Metabolic Blowtorch Diet Difference

Most fasting protocols will require you to fast for 16 hours, keeping any eating that you do within a specific 8 hour span of the day. Typically, this means that from the point you wake up in the morning, all your meals will fit into the first 8 hours. Then, you can't eat anything for the next 16 hours. However, the Metabolic Blowtorch Diet changes things around a little.

For one thing, the Metabolic Blowtorch Diet is split into two types of intermittent fasting timing: for men and for women. Men must fast for 16 to 20 hours per day. Women, on the other hand, must fast for only 12 to 15 hours per day. These hours are meant only for non-training days. When you're working out, fasting is not required. In fact, it's discouraged. The diet works with food, adjusting carbs on weight training days, instead of denying the body of the energy and recovery tools it needs to excel during and after workouts.

Does the Metabolic Blowtorch Diet Work?

The Metabolic Blowtorch Diet involves a certain learning curve. Moreover, it requires quite a substantial lifestyle change for the majority of users. That said, for those who stick to the strategy over a stretch of time, the reviews have been primarily positive. People like the way it provides the benefits of intermittent fasting, but not on training days when there is the potential to do more harm than good. It uses carb adjustments to compensate for the lack of fasting.

Many people also like that there is a version for both men and women, taking both types of metabolism into consideration. That said, it is important to point out that the Metabolic Blowtorch Diet is not a long-term dieting strategy. This is not the type of thing that you will be able to stick to for the rest of your life but is more appropriate for someone with specific fat loss and muscle building goals over a set length of time.

WEIGHT LOSS MEAL PLAN

This is probably the most important part of your meal prep routine. Prepping food alone won't necessarily help you drop pounds if you aren't following the basic steps for weight loss. Start with the following, in this order:

Calculate how many calories you need to lose weight here.

Get your macros on point using this.

And read this to learn the best foods for weight loss.

Complete with food lists, menu planning templates and expert advice to help you save time and money in the process.

Sensible Portions

Once you've got the basics down, it's time to start putting it into action.

Calories and macros go hand in hand, which is why meal prepping on a macro diet can make keeping your portion control in check and calorie control even easier -

especially since counting macros means you have an idea of how much of each type of food your should be eating.

You may also want to consider buying a food scale or use a food tracking app to be as precise as possible and learn the exact portion sizes that match your individual needs.

Keep in mind, the portions you use may change from one day to the next or one meal to the next, depending on your fitness and health goals. You can adjust your carb and protein portions around your workouts, eating more food when you are more active and a lighter meal on rest days or when you are not moving around as much.

Your carbohydrate needs are directly related to your level of physical activity, and you should eat more carbohydrates when you are the most active.

Here are some easy ways you can automatically get more nutrition and sensible portions into your meals:

Load up on veggies. They should make up 1/3 to 1/2 of your meal to provide high amounts of nutrients and fiber that will help keep your appetite in check and metabolism going strong.

Pick lean proteins to balance out the dish like chicken, fish, grass-fed beef, or tofu. Minimize breaded and fried versions to keep your calories in check. Eating more protein will help keep you satisfied and supports lean muscle, which is important for weight management.

Use whole grains like quinoa, farro, brown rice and whole grain pasta as a base. They travel well and pair with just about any protein, veggies, and flavor you add. You can also use beans, lentils, peas, corn or potatoes. Aim to keep your starch portion to 1/3 or less of your meal.

Cook with small amounts of healthy fats like olive oil and avocado oil, or top with whole fats like olives, nuts, and avocados. A little bit goes a long way, so keep your portions small and only add what you need for flavor.

Minimize added ingredients like salt, cheese, heavy sauces, high sugar dressings, etc. These can wrack up extra calories quickly from sugar and fat. Instead pile on calorie-free additions to add more flavor and variety - like lemon, fresh herbs, garlic, paprika, or chili flakes. Or choose lighter options like salsa, kimchi, nutritional yeast, and sugar-free dressings.

Portion Peanut Butter
WEIGHING YOUR FOOD

Learning how to weigh your food using a food scale is the most accurate way to control your portions. Even if you are using measuring cups and spoons, this still requires some eyeballing.

If you are new to meal prep or need to be super strict about your calories, consider using weights instead. Minor differences can really add up, especially when looking at high fat toppings, dressing and cooking oil.

For examples, 1 ounce vs. 1.5 ounces of cheese topping can look pretty similar, but the larger portion adds 43 calories, 3g protein, and 3g fat to your meal. This amount may seem minor, but if this happened twice a day, 5 days a week, you'd be adding almost 500 extra calories without realizing it.

WEIGHT LOSS

Weight loss can change your whole character. That always amazed me: Shedding pounds does change your personality. It changes your philosophy of life because you recognize that you are capable of using your mind to change your body.

The body weight is a sum of your muscle mass, fat mass, body water and also bone mass. Losing weight can sometimes backfire if not supported with a proper diet. Crash diets and other shortcuts may lead to a loss in muscle mass instead of fat mass. It may show fast results in the beginning, but your weight will shoot right back up the moment you leave exercising.

FAT LOSS

It is important that your workout adds muscle mass too. Too much body fat stores unwanted water and calories which makes you feel out of shape. However, some amount of fat is required for the absorption of fat-soluble vitamins and provide a cushioning to internal organs. Be regular with your exercise and reduce the number of calories you consume to make sure you lose fat mass.

Signs that you are losing muscle mass

If you do not substitute your workout with a proper diet or take to diets and shortcuts to lose weight, it can cause you to lose muscle mass instead of fat. Here are a few signs that you are losing muscle mass –

Regular workouts feel harder to complete

You feel sluggish throughout the day

Lower endurance

You have poor balance

You weight is stuck at one point

Here is how you can ensure that you do not lose out on the important muscle mass and get rid of only the fat in the body.

Exercising is not the only solution

It is important to maintain a proper diet when you have a regular workout routine. Eating less is not the answer. Instead, eat a balanced diet that gives the body enough nutrition to help muscles recover after your workout. If you do not eat well, you may lose muscle strength and eventually lose muscle mass as well.

Protein is very important

You must consume some form of protein in every meal. It's easy to complete your protein intake with eggs for breakfast or meat, cottage cheese, nuts and seeds throughout the day. It is important that you replace the protein that your muscles lose every day.

Don't cut carbs

Do not cut on carbs completely. Instead, keep an eye on refined or processed carbs. You can substitute them with whole grains like ragi, bajra or jowar. Carbohydrates are your steady source of energy.

Balance cardio and strength training

High-intensity interval training offers better results instead of long cardio activities. They add to muscle mass. You can also try and add weight training to help you maintain muscle mass. It is necessary that you take a day's rest from your workout to help your muscles time to rest and recover.

FACTS YOU NEED TO KNOW ABOUT WEIGHT LOSS.

Weight is more than fat (focus on body fat)

First and most importantly, getting that body you want is about more than just weight loss.In fact, weight is too general of a thing to focus on if you're really serious about getting fitter because it involves several factors including the amount of muscle in your body and water weight.

Assuming you're doing some sort of strength training, muscle is crucial. That's because muscle is heavier than fat, so by losing fat and gaining an equivalent amount of muscle you'd actually be gaining weight. However, your body would look slimmer and leaner than ever. Focus on body fat percentage (25-28% for women and 12-15% for men is the general recommendation, but check with your doctor) for a more accurate reading of whether your diet and exercise efforts are working.

Drop the wrong kind of calories, get enough of the right ones

Weight loss is all about calories. Most importantly, you need to know what different macronutrients count as calories and what each one does to your body. For example, white carbohydrates like bread and rice have a huge number of calories that provide little value to our body nutrition-wise. However, protein and certain types of fat are critical for your overall health.

All of the above count as calories when consumed, but the difference in your diet– and weight loss results– can be huge depending on how many of each you consume.

Track your food intake

Rolling off of the last point, you need to start watching your food intake like you watch for news of the next season of Stranger Things. Every single day, you need to track what you're consuming and how much you're consuming of it all. Everyone's body is different, so your number of calories and the right balance of macronutrients will be unique to you.

However, generally, you want to consume just under your recommended daily caloric intake. This will make your body start burning fat so that it can maintain its necessary energy consumption level (because it needs to get it from somewhere and it will turn first to your fat store).

Sleep can actually help you lose weight; The Science Behind a Good Night's Sleep

As with quite literally everything else tied to your physical and mental health, sleep is critical for weight loss. Why? Well, think of sleep as taking an ice bath if you were a professional athlete after a game. An ice bath helps heal the body after intense physical effort and sleep does the same for fat-burning after a long day and, especially, a good workout. Sleep is a time for everything in the body to recharge and optimize itself, including when most of the fat and general calorie-burning processes take place, so by getting enough sleep you're giving your body the time it needs to drop those inches.

Make healthy food convenient (and junk food not)
Weight loss needs to accompany lifestyle changes, otherwise, you'll too easily shift back into your old patterns and return to your original weight. One of the most important things to do along those lines is to make your diet-friendly foods the easiest and most convenient things for you to get a hold of, while sweets and other junk food should be thrown in a cupboard, moved behind your healthy snacks in the fridge, and so on.

You don't need to rid yourself of them entirely. In fact, doing so can hurt your weight loss efforts as you'll see later, but you do need to reduce the risk of those temptations while increasing the likelihood of choosing another healthier option.

Ditch the scale

Staring at a scale every day can be downright demoralizing. That's because our weight fluctuates throughout each day regularly whether we're working to lose weight or not. Part of this is because of the water content in our body, part of it the inverse relationship between body fat loss and muscle gain, as well as other regular bodily fluctuations.

In other words: don't look at the scale every single day and don't look at it just once in a single day. Preferably, you stay off the scale and go based on body fat percentage and how you feel. However, if you really want to look at the scale, then do it weekly and look at it a few times in that day to get a better average weight.

Weight loss pills are a bad, bad idea

I know, the idea of a magical weight loss pill making your fat dissolve away like a dream is enticing. But, alas, it's too good to be true (if that wasn't obvious already).

Here's an idea of some of the side effects of weight loss pills:

- Pulmonary hypertension (potentially fatal)
- Heart disease
- Increase blood pressure
- Increased heart rate
- Insomnia
- Dizziness
- Restlessness

Weight loss pills often promise immediate results. However, they do nothing to change your diet or physical exercise habits, ability to resist temptation, and all the other habits that made your body the weight it is now. So, even if do manage to get past the nasty side effects and get results, you'll eventually end up back where you started. To create a real, lasting change, you need to change your fitness and nutrition habits.

You can't just keep cutting calories

I know what you might be thinking then. "I want results fast, so I'll just cut calories drastically and get there quicker." After all, the math basically adds up. Starving yourself with too few calories is a no-no, so don't even think of trying to fast-track your diet by eating air. Unfortunately, it just doesn't work that way.

By starving yourself, you can cause your body to turn catabolic, a state where your body essentially starts eating muscle instead of fat to maintain itself. That can then have all kinds of bad side effects on your body. So, yeah, no starving.

Apple cider vinegar is disgusting. You should probably drink it.

Apple cider vinegar is a wonder elixir purportedly with the ability to lower blood sugar, cholesterol and aid in weight loss among other things. It's positively disgusting, however, if you're serious about shedding some pounds, try having a little of it each day. Most recommendations say two teaspoons a day in water or tea. And feel free to throw some honey in there to take some of the edge off.

A cheat day is a must (but not for the reason you're thinking)

You've probably heard of a cheat day before: a day where, pinned between memories of a strict, painful diet and the dread of a difficult week filled with boring, lifeless meals, is a shimmer of hope that you can consume whatever you want and in whatever quantity. For this one day, you have total freedom. Want to get those cupcakes you saw earlier this week at the store.

However, what most people aren't aware of is a cheat day has an entirely different and even more critical role in a diet: to maintain metabolic rate. Here's the thing: your new diet has the potential to slow down your metabolism because you'll be consuming fewer calories. When this happens, you'll burn fewer calories and your weight loss quota will be that much harder to hit.

But by having one day in the week where you go wild, you're telling the body that it needs to maintain its current metabolic rate, maximizing your weight loss efforts all week long and enjoying yourself in the process.

Meal prepping makes everything easiermeal-prepping

Seriously, sticking to a strict diet is not only critical for weight loss it's downright draining. It takes a lot of work to put together a diet that can help you lose weight, however, it's worth it.

And taking the time to prep those meals beforehand each week makes it exponentially easier to stick to that diet because you've removed any sort of resistance to it, making it easier just to eat what is already in front of you rather than going to grab or make something else.

Use HIIT (and strength training)

It's important to work out if you're really serious about losing weight, however, it's not good enough to just throw on one of those old Jazzercise videos and get moving (as much as I know you like them). Research has proven the benefits of HIIT or high-intensity interval training are far greater than your average workout for both cardio and weight training, both important parts of a complete weight loss regimen (cardio drops calories and keeps your heart healthy, strength training helps burn fat).

With HIIT, you can get the same benefit in fifteen minutes what you'd get in one hour of a typical workout.

Drop the weekend drinks couple
As sad-happy as it might sound to some, dropping alcohol can immediately result in dropping pounds. Most people aren't aware of just how many calories are in their favorite drinks, sometimes even more than sugary sodas, so by dropping alcohol or reducing your intake, you can make some much-needed progress fast.

Don't blame it on your thyroid

Growing up, I had a friend with a thyroid problem. She was a bit hefty as a child, but, once the issue was discovered all that excess weight disappeared and never came back. As promising as this sounds, she's a minority. For most people, women being the more common case, this isn't the issue. And, by trying to look for other reasons why you might not be the weight you'd like to be, you're just giving yourself excuses. Be realistic but also be honest with yourself.

More water, less Starbucksgirl, forming habit of drinking water

In addition to alcohol, many of the other drinks we consume regularly have huge amounts of calories. This includes:

- Soda
- Juice
- Lattes / similar Starbucks-like drinks

The thing is, as opposed to the kinds of necessary calories we talked about earlier, like protein and good fats, these are empty calories that simply fill us up and make us gain weight. In other words, we don't need them.

Instead, drink lots of water, which doesn't just help you cut the calories but helps your body's various processes run smoothly, which can help assist in weight loss.

It's less what you're consuming and more about over consuming

If you think sugar, alcohol, gluten, or some other kind of food or drink is making you fat, guess again. Sure, each of these plays a part, however, it's less about what individual things you're consuming and more about how much you're consuming. Overeating is what results in weight gain (more calories than our body needs to operate), so if you cut back on your Starbucks, lower your alcohol consumption, and reduce the number of times you eat at Pepe's in a month, you can keep all of the things you like while drastically reducing your calorie count and shedding some weight.

Everyone's body is different

This is easily one of the most important points to keep in mind. At one point or another, we all hear that XYZ celebrity, friend, or family member did some specific diet that worked wonders for them. The thing is, everyone's body is different and there's more of a likelihood that same method won't work for you, so pay attention to your own body, and find what works for you.

There are no quick fixes; Morning exercise is one of the most powerful ways to start your day

There are things you can do to lose a bit of weight quickly (like dropping alcohol), however, it's important to keep in mind that there are zero quick fixes to real, significant weight loss. Don't pay any mind to any celebrity fad diet, they're just playing to the impatient masses. You need to be willing to exercise more than just your body to lose weight. You need to exercise your patience.

Make it a lifestyle

The final and possibly most important thing of all to know is this: healthy living, whether it's dropping a few pounds now, a lot of pounds over the next year, building muscle, or something else, needs to be made a lifestyle. This is more mental than anything else, but it has a profound effect on your ability to remain consistent in your effort, the prime adversary in any endeavor, including losing weight

PATHS TO IMPROVED DIET OF WEIGHT LOSS

Nutrition

In general, eat fewer calories than your body uses in order to lose weight. Calories come from the foods you eat and drink. Some foods have more calories than others. For example, foods that are high in fat and sugar are high in calories, too. Some foods are made up of "empty calories." These add a lot of calories to your diet without providing nutritional value.

If you eat more calories than your body uses, your body stores them as fat. One pound of fat is about 3,500 calories. To lose 1 pound of fat in a week, you have to eat 3,500 fewer calories. That divides out to 500 fewer calories a day. One thing you can do is remove regular soda from your diet. This alone cuts over 350 calories per day. You also can burn off 3,500 more calories a week. You can do this by exercising or being more active. Most people do a combination of the two. If you do this for 7 days, you can lose 1 pound of fat in a week.

Most experts believe that you should not lose more than 2 pounds per week. This can mean that you are losing water weight and lean muscle mass instead of stored fat. It can leave you with less energy and cause you to gain the weight back. Try taking a food habits survey. It will tell you where you need to make changes to your diet. It also can identify what nutrients you lack. Tips for improving your diet include:

Only eat when you are hungry. This could mean 3 meals and 1 snack every day. Or it may mean 5 to 6 small meals throughout the day. If you aren't hungry, don't eat. Don't skip meals. Skipping meals on purpose does not lead to weight loss. It can make you feel hungrier later on. It could cause you to overeat or make poor food choices. Wait 15 minutes before getting a second helping of food. It can take this long for your body to process whether it's still hungry. Try to eat a variety of whole foods. This includes lean meats, whole grains, and dairy. When choosing fruits and vegetables, eat the rainbow.

Avoid processed foods and foods high in fat or sugar. Drink plenty of fluids. Choose no- or low-calorie drinks, like water or unsweetened tea. In some cases, your doctor may refer you to a nutrition specialist. They can help you with grocery shopping and recipes that fit your needs.

Exercise
Both adults and children should get regular physical activity. It is important for losing weight and maintaining good health. Below are ways to increase your activity and burn calories.

Add 10 minutes a day to your current exercise routine.

Challenge yourself. Move from moderate to intense activities.

Take the stairs instead of the elevator.

Park further away or walk to your destination instead of driving.

Do more household chores, such as dusting, vacuuming, or weeding.

Go for a walk or run with your dog and/or kids.

Exercise at home while watching TV.

Be active on your vacations. Try going for a hike or bike ride.

Buy a pedometer or activity tracker. This measures how many steps you take each day. Try to increase your daily number of steps over time. (You can buy pedometers at sporting goods stores.) Some experts recommend walking at least 10,000 steps a day.

Limit time spent online, watching TV, and playing video games. This should equal less than 2 hours total per day.

Moderate activity;

Approximate calories per 30 minutes

Stretching

90

Light weight lifting

110

Walking (3.5 miles per hour, or mph)

140

Bicycling (less than 10 mph)

145

Light yard work or gardening

165

Golf

165

Dancing

165

Hiking

185

Intense activity;

Approximate calories per 30 minutes

Heavy weight lifting

220

Heavy yard work

220

Basketball

220

Walking (4.5 mph)

230

Aerobics

240

Swimming (freestyle laps)

255

Running or jogging (5 mph, or 12 minutes/mile)

295

Bicycling (more than 10 mph)

295

Average calories burned for a person who weighs 154 pounds. If you weigh more, you will burn more calories. If you weigh less, you will burn fewer calories.

Lifestyle

You may have to alter your schedule to make changes to your diet and exercise. This could mean waking up early to work out or packing your lunch so you don't eat fast food. Along with diet and exercise, you should make other lifestyle changes. Getting enough sleep can help you lose weight. Sleep affects your body's hormones. This includes the hormones that tell your body if it is hungry or full. You also should try to reduce your stress level. A lot of people relate stress to weight gain.

Things to consider

When you start a weight loss plan, there are things to keep in mind. You may have an obstacle that makes it hard to lose weight. Or it could have led to weight gain in the first place. You also need to be careful of where you get advice. Your weight loss plan should be safe and successful.

Medical conditions that contribute to obesity

For a some people, weight gain can be related to genetics. Others may have a medical condition that makes it hard to lose weight. Examples of this include:

- Hormonal disorders
- Cushing's disease
- Diabetes
- Hypothyroidism
- Polycystic ovarian syndrome (PCOS)
- Sleep disorders
- Obstructive sleep apnea
- Upper airway respiratory syndrome
- Eating disorders
- Bulimia

- Carbohydrate craving syndrome.
- Certain medicines also can interfere with your weight loss efforts. This includes:
- Antihistamines for allergies.
- Alpha or beta blockers for high blood pressure.
- Insulin or sulfonylureas for diabetes.
- Progestins for birth control.
- Tricyclic antidepressants for depression.
- Lithium for manic depression.
- Valproate for epilepsy.
- Neuroleptics for schizophrenia.

Talk to your doctor about how to manage your weight despite these obstacles. Lifestyle changes, treatment, or surgery can help. You also may benefit from a support group or counseling.

Diet pills, supplements, and fad diets
Some companies and people claim diet pills make you lose weight. This may be true at first, but pills don't help you keep the weight off. They don't teach you how to make lifestyle changes. The U.S. Food and Drug

Administration (FDA) does not test most diet pills. Many of them can have harmful side effects. Talk to your doctor if you think you need a supplement. They can recommend one that doesn't interact with your medicines or conditions.

Fad diets also are not proven to be safe or help you lose weight. They often offer short-term changes, but don't help you keep the weight off. People who promote fad diets are famous or get paid to make claims. This does not make them correct or trustworthy. There is no one magic diet that helps every person lose weight. The idea of "going on a diet" implies that you will "go off the diet" one day. Do not rely on a fad diet to do the work for you. Instead, find a healthy, balanced eating plan that can become a practical lifestyle.

WEIGHT-LOSS MANAGEMENT

There are tools you can use throughout your weight loss plan. They help to track your progress and reach your goals. These include:

- A pedometer to count your steps.
- A food diary, or journal.
- Smartphone apps to record diet and exercise.
- A measuring tape or scale.
- A BMI calculator.

Rules Of Weight Loss That Lasts Before You Start

Before you even begin to attack a weight-loss plan, it pays to remember this: You are not fat. You have fat. Losing weight isn't about blame or shame; it's simply another achievement to accomplish, like training for a race or finally cranking out 10 push-ups. "Dieting is like any other skill you have to buckle down and work at it, the diet program coordinator at the Beck Institute for Cognitive Behavior Therapy and a coauthor of The Diet Trap Solution. As long as you act in a smart, reasonable way, you'll ultimately get where you want to be.

To help you reach your goal weight and maintain it, we examined the latest research and talked to top experts to compile the 10 tenets for weight loss that have been proved to deliver results.

It's Not a Diet. It's a Lifestyle

Thinking of a diet as something you're on and suffering through only for the short term doesn't work. To shed weight and keep it off, you need to make permanent changes to the way you eat. It's OK to indulge occasionally, of course, but if you cut calories temporarily and then revert to your old way of eating, you'll gain back the weight quicker than you can say

Research shows that one of the best predictors of long-term weight loss is how many pounds you drop in the first month. It makes sense: Immediate results are motivating. For that reason, nutritionists often suggest being stricter for the first two weeks of your new eating strategy to build momentum. Cut out added sugar and alcohol and avoid unrefined carbs. "After that, ease small amounts of those foods back into your diet for a plan you can live with for the long term.

There's a Right Way to Exercise

Working out burns calories and fat and boosts your metabolism by building muscle. But those trying to lose weight are notorious for overestimating the number of calories they burn and underestimating the amount they take in. Unfortunately, your system is biologically programmed to hold on to extra pounds. That means when you start exercising, your body senses the deficit and ramps up its hunger signals, according to a review of weight-loss studies. If you're not diligent, you'll eat everything you burn and then some.

Cardio gets all the exercise glory, but strength and interval training are the real heroes. They help you build lean muscle, which in turn increases your metabolism and calorie-burning ability. Every week, strength-train two to three days. For the best results, also do three to five cardio sessions that burn 250 to 400 calories each.

Don't Overreact to Mild Hunger

Some women have a hard time losing weight because of hunger anxiety. To them, being hungry is bad something to be avoided at all costs so they carry snacks with them and eat when they don't need to, Alpert explains. Others eat because they're stressed out or bored. While you never want to get to the point of being ravenous (that's when bingeing is likely to happen), a hunger pang, a craving, or the fact that it's 3:00 p.m. should not send you racing for the vending machine or obsessing about the energy bar in your purse. Ideally, you should put off eating until your stomach is growling and it's difficult to concentrate.

When you feel the urge to eat, use the HALT method. Ask yourself, Am I really hungry? Or am I angry or anxious, lonely or bored, or tired? If you're still not certain, try the apple test. "If you're truly hungry, an apple should seem delicious; if it doesn't, something else is going on. In that case, give yourself a pep talk instead of a snack. "If hunger isn't the problem, food isn't the solution. There are a lot of other ways to deal with boredom or anxiety like going for a walk, hitting the gym, or texting a friend and those things have zero negative consequences.

Not All Calories Are Created Equal

The mechanics of weight loss are pretty simple: Take in fewer calories than you use for energy. But the kind of food you eat makes all the difference. "A calorie is not just a calorie. Processed food that's high in saturated fat and refined starch or sugar can cause inflammation that disrupts the hormone signals that tell your brain you're full, he explains. The result: You eat a lot more. Plus, studies show that junk food can be addictive; the more you eat it, the more you need to get the same feel-good effects. "One handful of potato chips won't cut it any longer, so you keep eating and eating.

Clean up your diet. Swap in whole, unprocessed foods, including vegetables, lean protein, and healthy fats that will fill you up and give you the biggest nutritional bang for your calorie buck. In a few weeks, as your brain starts receiving regular hunger and fullness signals once again, you'll notice that you feel less hungry overall and naturally start cutting back on the amount you eat.

While you're at it, log each meal. Keeping a daily food diary (there are tons of apps for this) leads to significant weight loss because it makes you accountable, research shows. One study published in the American Journal of Preventive Medicine found that people who kept daily food records lost about twice as much weight as those who didn't.

Protein, Produce, and Plant-Based Fats Are Your Weight-Loss Trinity

Protein fills you up. You need it to build lean muscle, which keeps your metabolism humming so that you can torch more fat. People in a weight-loss program who ate double the recommended daily allowance for protein (about 110 grams for a 150-pound woman) lost 70 percent of their weight from fat, while people who ate the RDA lost only about 40 percent, one study found.

Produce is packed with filling fiber. "It's very difficult to consume too many calories if you're eating a lot of vegetables. Three cups of broccoli is a lot of food, yet only 93 calories. (Fruit is another story. It can be easy to overeat and can contain a lot of calories from sugar, so be sure to monitor your intake.

Plant-based fats like olive oil and those in avocados and nuts are healthy and extra satiating. Low-fat diets make people irritable and feel deprived because fat tastes good and keeps you full. Aim to incorporate each of the three Ps into every meal and snack. People who eat protein throughout the day are able to keep weight off, according to a study in the American Journal of Clinical Nutrition. In addition to meat, poultry and seafood, good sources are beans, lentils, eggs, tofu, and yogurt. As for fat, keep portion sizes in check by measuring out salad dressing, oil, and nut butters (shoot for one to two tablespoons). Finally, eat veggies or a little fruit at every meal. People who did that consumed 308 fewer calories but didn't feel any hungrier than when they didn't eat more produce, a study in the journal Appetite noted.

Meal Skipping, Juice Fasts, and Crash Diets Will Backfire. Always

When you lose weight on a fast or a crash diet, you don't learn to eat healthier, adjust your portion sizes, or deal with whatever is triggering your overeating in the first place, so the pounds quickly return. The physical damage goes deeper. "The worse the quality of a diet or the more restrictive it is, the more you end up burning precious muscle to supply energy. You're losing muscle instead of fat, so the weight loss is just an illusion of success. Depending on how much weight you need to drop and how much you currently eat, try to cut 500 to 1,000 calories a day through both diet and exercise, Frutchey advises. Limiting yourself to about 1,500 calories a day won't leave you starving, but it will help you see motivating changes on the scale.

How You Eat Is As Important As What You Eat

In order for your brain to register that you're full, you need to focus on what you're eating. Physical satiety is closely tied to psychological satisfaction. People tell me all the time how difficult it is for them to lose weight because they love to eat, yet they never concentrate on their food—they eat while watching TV, reading, driving, and working." No wonder that, according to research, eating when you're distracted results in consuming a significant number of extra calories a day.

Sit down whenever you eat, preferably at a table. "If you ask someone to recall what she ate in a day, she'll forget most of the food she consumed standing up. Turn off the TV or computer, put down your phone, and look at your food. Smell it. Chew slowly, and don't put another bite on your fork until you swallow. When women ate lunch this attentively, they consumed 30 percent less when snacking later than those who listened to an audiobook at lunchtime, according to a study in the British Journal of Nutrition.

Weighing Yourself Really Works
The scale provides the best evidence about whether your efforts are paying off. Seeing the numbers tick up or down or stagnate is motivation to keep going—or to rethink your approach. A 2015 study at Cornell University found that daily weigh-ins helped people lose

more weight, keep it off, and maintain that loss, even after two years.

Step on the scale at the same time every day for the best results. If your weight shoots up several pounds from one weigh-in to the next, don't freak out. Eating a lot of salt the night before or having your period is the likely culprit. The number should return to normal in a day or two. It's a steady climb that you need to do something about.

Too Much Stress and Too Little Sleep Are Your Enemies

When you're tired and frazzled, your body cranks up the production of cortisol, the stress hormone that can cause carb cravings. Not getting enough sleep also boosts your levels of ghrelin, a hormone associated with hunger, while suppressing leptin, a hormone that signals fullness and satiety. People on a diet who slept only five and a half hours a night for two weeks lost 55 percent less fat and were hungrier than those who slept eight and a half hours, according to a study in the Canadian Medical Association Journal

Prioritize sleep, aiming for seven hours or more a night, which research shows helps lower stress. And make sure you're getting quality. If a snoring spouse or a fidgety cat wakes you up frequently throughout the night, you may end up getting the equivalent of just four hours of sleep, according to a study from Tel Aviv University. Keep pets out of the bedroom, and use a white-noise app to drown out snoring

You Will Hit a Plateau And You Can Bust Through It

As you slim down, your body releases much less leptin, the fullness hormone. "If you lose 10 percent of your body weight, leptin drops by about 50 percent. "Your brain is programmed to think you've shed more pounds than you actually have, and it tells your body it needs more food and should burn fewer calories." That's why plateaus happen and what makes maintaining weight loss so difficult. In addition, when you're lighter, you require fewer calories for energy. "You might have burned 100 calories taking a walk before, but now your body needs only 80 calories to go the same distance.

We'll reiterate: If you're not strength training, start right now. Building muscle can raise your metabolism to help you overcome a plateau. To keep your body challenged and burning calories, incorporate new moves and more intense intervals into your workouts or add another sweat session to your weekly routine. Alternatively, cut an extra 100 calories or so a day from your diet. Now that you've lost weight, your body simply doesn't need as much fuel. Still stuck? Try eating carbs last at every meal, after your protein and vegetables. Research shows that doing so will reduce your blood sugar by almost 40 percent. Blood sugar influences weight he explains, so this strategy could help.

Popular Weight Loss Strategies

Cut calories

Some experts believe that successfully managing your weight comes down to a simple equation: If you eat fewer calories than you burn, you lose weight. Sounds easy, right? Then why is losing weight so hard?

Weight loss isn't a linear event over time. When you cut calories, you may drop weight for the first few weeks, for example, and then something changes. You eat the same number of calories but you lose less weight or no weight at all. That's because when you lose weight you're losing water and lean tissue as well as fat, your metabolism slows, and your body changes in other ways. So, in order to continue dropping weight each week, you need to continue cutting calories.

A calorie isn't always a calorie. Eating 100 calories of high fructose corn syrup, for example, can have a different effect on your body than eating 100 calories of broccoli. The trick for sustained weight loss is to ditch the foods that are packed with calories but don't make you feel full (like candy) and replace them with foods that fill you up without being loaded with calories (like vegetables). Many of us don't always eat simply to satisfy hunger. We also turn to food for comfort or to relieve stress which can quickly derail any weight loss plan.

Cut carbs

A different way of viewing weight loss identifies the problem as not one of consuming too many calories, but rather the way the body accumulates fat after consuming carbohydrates in particular the role of the hormone insulin. When you eat a meal, carbohydrates from the food enter your bloodstream as glucose. In order to keep your blood sugar levels in check, your body always burns off this glucose before it burns off fat from a meal.

If you eat a carbohydrate-rich meal (lots of pasta, rice, bread, or French fries, for example), your body releases insulin to help with the influx of all this glucose into your blood. As well as regulating blood sugar levels, insulin does two things: It prevents your fat cells from releasing fat for the body to burn as fuel (because its priority is to burn off the glucose) and it creates more fat cells for storing everything that your body can't burn off. The result is that you gain weight and your body now requires more fuel to burn, so you eat more. Since insulin only burns carbohydrates, you crave carbs and so begins a vicious cycle of consuming carbs and gaining weight. To lose weight, the reasoning goes, you need to break this cycle by reducing carbs.

Most low-carb diets advocate replacing carbs with protein and fat, which could have some negative long-term effects on your health. If you do try a low-carb diet, you can reduce your risks and limit your intake of saturated and trans fats by choosing lean meats, fish and vegetarian sources of protein, low-fat dairy products, and eating plenty of leafy green and non-starchy vegetables.

Cut fat
It's a mainstay of many diets: if you don't want to get fat, don't eat fat. Walk down any grocery store aisle and you'll be bombarded with reduced-fat snacks, dairy, and packaged meals. But while our low-fat options have

exploded, so have obesity rates. So, why haven't low-fat diets worked for more of us?

Not all fat is bad. Healthy or "good" fats can actually help to control your weight, as well as manage your moods and fight fatigue. Unsaturated fats found in avocados, nuts, seeds, soy milk, tofu, and fatty fish can help fill you up, while adding a little tasty olive oil to a plate of vegetables, for example, can make it easier to eat healthy food and improve the overall quality of your diet. We often make the wrong trade-offs. Many of us make the mistake of swapping fat for the empty calories of sugar and refined carbohydrates. Instead of eating whole-fat yoghurt, for example, we eat low- or no-fat versions that are packed with sugar to make up for the loss of taste. Or we swap our fatty breakfast bacon for a muffin or donut that causes rapid spikes in blood sugar.

Follow the Mediterranean diet
The Mediterranean diet emphasizes eating good fats and good carbs along with large quantities of fresh fruits and vegetables, nuts, fish, and olive oil—and only modest amounts of meat and cheese. The Mediterranean diet is

more than just about food, though. Regular physical activity and sharing meals with others are also major components. Whatever weight loss strategy you try, it's important to stay motivated and avoid common dieting pitfalls, such as emotional eating.

Control emotional eating

We don't always eat simply to satisfy hunger. All too often, we turn to food when we're stressed or anxious, which can wreck any diet and pack on the pounds. Do you eat when you're worried, bored, or lonely? Do you snack in front of the TV at the end of a stressful day? Recognizing your emotional eating triggers can make all the difference in your weight-loss efforts. If you eat when you're:

Stressed – find healthier ways to calm yourself. Try yoga, meditation, or soaking in a hot bath.

Low on energy – find other mid-afternoon pick-me-ups. Try walking around the block, listening to energizing music, or taking a short nap.

Lonely or bored – reach out to others instead of reaching for the refrigerator. Call a friend who makes you laugh, take your dog for a walk, or go to the library, mall, or park—anywhere there's people.

Practice mindful eating instead

Avoid distractions while eating. Try not to eat while working, watching TV, or driving. It's too easy to mindlessly overeat. Pay attention. Eat slowly, savoring the smells and textures of your food. If your mind wanders, gently return your attention to your food and how it tastes.

Mix things up to focus on the experience of eating. Try using chopsticks rather than a fork, or use your utensils with your non-dominant hand.

Stop eating before you are full. It takes time for the signal to reach your brain that you've had enough. Don't feel obligated to always clean your plate.

Stay motivated

Permanent weight loss requires making healthy changes to your lifestyle and food choices. To stay motivated:

Find a cheering section. Social support means a lot. Programs like Jenny Craig and Weight Watchers use group support to impact weight loss and lifelong healthy eating. Seek out support whether in the form of family, friends, or a support group to get the encouragement you need.

Slow and steady wins the race. Losing weight too fast can take a toll on your mind and body, making you feel sluggish, drained, and sick. Aim to lose one to two pounds a week so you're losing fat rather than water and muscle.

Set goals to keep you motivated. Short-term goals, like wanting to fit into a bikini for the summer, usually don't work as well as wanting to feel more confident or become healthier for your children's sakes. When temptation strikes, focus on the benefits you'll reap from being healthier.

Use tools to track your progress. Smartphone apps, fitness trackers, or simply keeping a journal can help you keep track of the food you eat, the calories you burn, and the weight you lose. Seeing the results in black and white can help you stay motivated.

Get plenty of sleep. Lack of sleep stimulates your appetite so you want more food than normal; at the same time, it stops you feeling satisfied, making you want to keep eating. Sleep deprivation can also affect your motivation, so aim for eight hours of quality sleep a night.

Cut down on sugar and refined carbs

Whether or not you're specifically aiming to cut carbs, most of us consume unhealthy amounts of sugar and refined carbohydrates such as white bread, pizza dough, pasta, pastries, white flour, white rice, and sweetened breakfast cereals. Replacing refined carbs with their whole-grain counterparts and eliminating candy and desserts is only part of the solution, though. Sugar is hidden in foods as diverse as canned soups and vegetables, pasta sauce, margarine, and many reduced fat foods. Since your body gets all it needs from sugar naturally occurring in food, all this added sugar amounts to nothing but a lot of empty calories and unhealthy spikes in your blood glucose.

Less sugar can mean a slimmer waistline
Calories obtained from fructose (found in sugary beverages such as soda and processed foods like doughnuts, muffins, and candy) are more likely to add to fat around your belly. Cutting back on sugary foods can mean a slimmer waistline as well as a lower risk of diabetes.

Fill up with fruit, veggies, and fiber
Even if you're cutting calories, that doesn't necessarily mean you have to eat less food. High-fiber foods such as fruit, vegetables, beans, and whole grains are higher in volume and take longer to digest, making them filling— and great for weight-loss.

It's generally okay to eat as much fresh fruit and non-starchy vegetables as you want you'll feel full before you've overdone it on the calories.

Eat vegetables raw or steamed, not fried or breaded, and dress them with herbs and spices or a little olive oil for flavor.

Add fruit to low sugar cereal—blueberries, strawberries, sliced bananas. You'll still enjoy lots of sweetness, but with fewer calories, less sugar, and more fiber.

Bulk out sandwiches by adding healthy veggie choices like lettuce, tomatoes, sprouts, cucumbers, and avocado.

Snack on carrots or celery with hummus instead of a high-calorie chips and dip.

Add more veggies to your favorite main courses to make your dish more substantial. Even pasta and stir-fries can be diet-friendly if you use less noodles and more vegetables.

Start your meal with salad or vegetable soup to help fill you up so you eat less of your entrée.

Take charge of your food environment

Set yourself up for weight-loss success by taking charge of your food environment: when you eat, how much you eat, and what foods you make easily available.

Cook your own meals at home. This allows you to control both portion size and what goes in to the food. Restaurant and packaged foods generally contain a lot more sugar, unhealthy fat, and calories than food cooked at home—plus the portion sizes tend to be larger.

Serve yourself smaller portions. Use small plates, bowls, and cups to make your portions appear larger. Don't eat out of large bowls or directly from food containers, which makes it difficult to assess how much you've eaten.

Eat early. Studies suggest that consuming more of your daily calories at breakfast and fewer at dinner can help you drop more pounds. Eating a larger, healthy breakfast can jump start your metabolism, stop you feeling hungry during the day, and give you more time to burn off the calories.

Fast for 14 hours a day. Try to eat dinner earlier in the day and then fast until breakfast the next morning. Eating only when you're most active and giving your digestion a long break may aid weight loss.

Plan your meals and snacks ahead of time. You can create your own small portion snacks in plastic bags or containers. Eating on a schedule will help you avoid eating when you aren't truly hungry.

Drink more water. Thirst can often be confused with hunger, so by drinking water you can avoid extra calories.

Limit the amount of tempting foods you have at home. If you share a kitchen with non-dieters, store indulgent foods out of sight.

Get moving
The degree to which exercise aids weight loss is open to debate, but the benefits go way beyond burning calories. Exercise can increase your metabolism and improve your outlook—and it's something you can benefit from right now. Go for a walk, stretch, move around and you'll

have more energy and motivation to tackle the other steps in your weight-loss program.

Lack time for a long workout? Three 10-minute spurts of exercise per day can be just as good as one 30-minute workout. Remember: anything is better than nothing. Start off slowly with small amounts of physical activity each day. Then, as you start to lose weight and have more energy, you'll find it easier to become more physically active.

Find exercise you enjoy. Try walking with a friend, dancing, hiking, cycling, playing Frisbee with a dog, enjoying a pickup game of basketball, or playing activity-based video games with your kids.

Keeping the Weight Off

You may have heard the widely quoted statistic that 95% of people who lose weight on a diet will regain it within a few years or even months. While there isn't much hard evidence to support that claim, it is true that many weight-loss plans fail in the long term. Often that's simply because diets that are too restrictive are very hard to maintain over time. However, that doesn't mean your weight loss attempts are doomed to failure.

Since it was established in 1994, The National Weight Control Registry (NWCR) in the United States, has tracked over 10,000 individuals who have lost significant amounts of weight and kept it off for long periods of time. The study has found that participants who've been successful in maintaining their weight loss share some common strategies. Whatever diet you use to lose weight in the first place, adopting these habits may help you to keep it off:

Stay physically active. Successful dieters in the NWCR study exercise for about 60 minutes, typically walking.

Keep a food log. Recording what you eat every day helps to keep you accountable and motivated.

Eat breakfast every day. Most commonly in the study, it's cereal and fruit. Eating breakfast boosts metabolism and staves off hunger later in the day.

Eat more fiber and less unhealthy fat than the typical American diet. Regularly check the scale. Weighing yourself weekly may help you to detect any small gains in weight, enabling you to promptly take corrective action before the problem escalates. Watch less television. Cutting back on the time spent sitting in front of a screen can be a key part of adopting a more active lifestyle and preventing weight gain.

We all strive and work hard to reach our ideal body weight. However, losing weight should not be the only goal of your weight loss regimen. Your body weight is not only ruled by the amount of fat, but also muscle mass, bone mass and metabolism. This is where the difference between weight loss and fat loss lies. Your workout should work on losing the extra fat in your body.

RAPID WEIGHT LOSS FOR WOMEN

So many marketers promise "fast weight loss" it's difficult to sort through them all.

Most rapid weight loss pitches fall into these categories:

Starvation Diets

Beyonce popularized the so-called "master cleanse" diet: water, lemon juice, maple syrup, and cayenne pepper. Variations of these diets have been around since at least the 1950s. They often also promise "detoxification" through colonics or enemas.

Diet Pills and Supplements

Dozens of diet supplements promise to speed weight loss. Generally, they claim either to block absorption of nutrients, increase metabolism, or burn fat.

Very Low-Calorie Diets (VLCDs)

One proven method of rapid weight loss is the medically supervised very low-calorie diet (VLCD). Most of what is known about rapid weight loss comes from studies of people on these diets.

Creams, Devices, and Magic Voodoo Spells

There seems to be no end to the dubious ideas promoted in the name of rapid weight loss. Most promise to replace diet or exercise.

Printed in Great Britain
by Amazon

26583176R00040